EXTREME BODY BUILDING AND FITNESS

BY

MICHAEL R. MASTERSON

DISCLAIMER

This data isn't introduced by a clinical professional and is for instructive and educational purposes as it were. The substance isn't expected to fill in for proficient clinical counsel, determination, or treatment. Continuously look for the guidance of your doctor or other qualified wellbeing suppliers with any inquiries you might have in regards to a clinical condition. Never dismiss proficient clinical counsel or defer in looking for it in light of something you have perused.

Since regular or potentially dietary enhancements are not FDA endorsed, they should be joined by a two-section disclaimer on the item name: that the assertion has not been assessed by FDA and that the item isn't planned to "analyze, treat, fix or forestall any illness. The creator and distributor of this course and the going with materials have involved their earnest attempts in setting up this course. The creator and distributor make no portrayal or guarantees regarding the precision, appropriateness, wellness, or culmination of the items in this course. The data contained in this course is stringently for instructive purposes. Thusly, in the event that you wish to apply thoughts contained in this course, you are assuming complete ownership of your activities.

The creator and distributor disavow any guarantees (express or inferred), merchantability, or readiness for a specific reason. The creator and distributor will on no occasion be held at risk to any party for any immediate, roundabout, corrective, extraordinary, accidental, or other significant harms emerging straightforwardly or by implication from any utilization of this material, which is if "with no guarantees", and without guarantees. As usual, the counsel of an able lawful, charge, bookkeeping, clinical or other experts ought to be looked for. The creator and distributor don't warrant the exhibition, adequacy, or appropriateness of any destinations recorded or connected to in this course.

TABLE OF CONTENTS

CHAPTER 1

WEIGHT TRAINING: TIPS FOR SUCCESS

There are two distinct approaches to starting a lifting weights system; the simple way and the hard way. Ypu can decide for yourself with the degree to which you will adhere to the system and consequently demonstrate a triumph. Since you have a decision you should set up a legitimate carved-out plan for yourself to choose the ideal choice. Assuming you are like me (and like a huge number of other savvy individuals everywhere) you will presumably decide to seek after the simple way, in which case you should begin with a strong exercise plan and get everythingbrecorded officially.

Setting up an exercise plan is in numerous ways tantamount to the kind of New Year goal arranging we as a whole will quite often do. The vast majority of us will generally surrender the goals in something like a day or two, yet here there is no surrendering. Guarantees are difficult to keep, essentially because a large portion will generally make troublesome commitments. The greater part of us tries not to stay by the goals we make toward the start of the year because our objectives are not practical. At the point when we vow to stop smoking in the new year, we disregard the way that surrendering smoking is a slow interaction and requirements time. So the shrewd method for quitting any pretense of smoking is smoking around 4 cigarettes every day, then, at that point, bring it down to 2, etc. There is no reason for hoping to quit any pretense of smoking very much like that just since we have vowed to.

Likewise, when you plan your weight training system remember that it needs a bunch of feasible objectives to truly work out. You won't transform into a Stallone in a month so don't plan to, give yourself a casual time-breaking point of saying a half year for that. Likewise, recollect when you are simply starting you won't have the sort of endurance an expert competitor or an encounter jock will have so don't get unsettled on the off chance that you can't stay aware of Arnie (who has been rehearsing for 2 years at this point) on your most memorable exercise meeting itself. Try not to make your rec center meeting a self-image tussle, you don't have anything to demonstrate anything here. Take time to unwind and pass judgment on your advancement cleverly.

At the point when you start your system hold it to something like 2 days in seven days. Ensure you have at least 2 hours in your grasp so you don't need to hustle through the exercise. Begin with a couple of cardio practices to energize your muscles. Invest a touch of energy on the treadmill or attempt some turning, anything that will siphon up your heart to around 80% of its typical limit is a great decision. Regardless of whether you believe that should start with cardiovascular activities ensure you do them after your activity system to assist your body with consuming more fat.

LIFTING WEIGHTS: WHEN TO START AND STOP

Weight training is an incredible method for chiseling your body into shape and losing those additional layers of fat. Preparing with loads can assist you with accelerating your digestion as well as fix and characterize your muscles to give you that ripped physique. While that sounds simple, however, don't be tricked into thinking that lifting weights is a stroll in the park. Lifting weights produces results (there are thousands of individuals all around the world who might handily vouch for that reality) gave you adhere to your system, remain restrained, and buckle down.

As we all who have attempted to get more fit sooner or later of time know losing the fat your body has put away after some time is difficult. It requires extraordinary commitment AND enormous work to offer its last farewell. This cycle itself can consume a large chunk of the day, thus the vast majority who take up weight training frequently become annoyed halfway and surrender it by and large. It's difficult to keep buckling down without seeing any impact of all your persistent effort on your body. Be that as it may, clearly the body finds an opportunity to respond and it won't be fast in answering because we need it to.

Remaining with the system requires enormous self-control, a specific measure of confidence, and the information in regards to when to stop working out. One of the absolute first things to learn in weight training is when to stop. Most working out novices will quite often continue to figure out till they nearly break down with fatigue. Presently, while propelling yourself is something to be thankful for getting out of hand is not. Everything occurs in its own benefit time, so regardless of how hard you train right on the main day it is impossible that you will see the impacts of that preparation right away. Likewise, serious activities right toward the start of the preparation can make you end up gravely stung.

Keep in mind, to keep your activity program fascinating you should guarantee that it's tomfoolery, or, more than likely you won't get back to it regularly and begin keeping away from it by certain means or others. Frequently weighty practicing can leave you feeling exhausted and expecting a break. Under such conditions do yourself some help and have some time off. Relax; a break will have only certain consequences for your body. It will utilize the time you spend away from the loads to recuperate its solidarity, what's more, begin fabricating new muscles, in this way guaranteeing that your re-visitation of the loads will be in a far better structure. Yet, that is not each a break from practicing will likewise leave you feeling sincerely loose and quiet.

Assuming you have quite recently begun working out you are likely yet to discover that your body benefits the most during the days when you stay inactive at home as opposed to siphoning the irons. This is because all the hard practice can leave your body feeling massively exhausted. The brief time frame off goes about as a kind of 'recuperation time' during which the muscles you pine for are made. Bulk doesn't increment during your exercise routine since muscles are excessively involved working then, at that point. All things considered, it extends in the days that follow your exercise. Hence, for the greatest advantage and absolute muscle building increment the time you spend away from the rec center and simply unwind, you will love the outcomes

CHAPTER 2

WEIGHT TRAINING: TIME MANAGEMENT

You could have started your weight training system however do you have a working-out plan? Indeed, such an arrangement ought to incorporate something beyond lifting a couple of extremely weighty irons, swallowing down some kelp, and getting a tan to look macho. Like all the other things the main rule in lifting weights also is to get an arrangement and get it down clearly. The subsequent rule is to adhere to this plan that you write down and attempt to achieve everything about covers as intently as you can.

One of the main pieces of your working-out plan ought to be how much time you dedicate to practicing ordinary, and how you figure out how to crush in that system between your different errands. In time usage we allude to steady exercises (that is the exercises you just HAVE to do during the recommended hours) as 'Large Rocks'. So exercises like express getting your girl from school or preparing lunch or a violin class is all Big Rocks since you need to do them when you need to.

So the initial step to making a weight training plan is denoting all such enormous rocks in your day to day plan. When those are very much checked essentially select the time among them and press in your activity system into them. Now that was simple, right? Well, it isn't the actual arrangement however staying on a course is the intense part. Attempt and be where you are supposed to be as indicated by your arrangement consistently. Don't be late, and don't invest additional energy on anything, even the rec center.

This carries us to the second piece of that significant exhortation: DO NOT invest energy superfluously, appreciating your chiseled physique before the mirror, or strutting around on the dance floor flaunting your recently ripped physique. It's valid, in all actuality do look cool doing those however you'd look much better assuming that you reclaimed the time you are squandering thusly and utilizing it at the rec center all things considered. It's difficult remaining roused and interruptions are wild, as in each field of life. To remain on track consequently read books or pay attention to CDs in regards to inspiration, using time effectively for achievement and contest. It's extraordinary, the sort of impact these have been known to have on individuals.

To update and further develop your lifting weights plan stay tuned to the Internet. Channel what you read, since most of the stuff you read online will undoubtedly be composed of genuinely idiotic, frantic wannabe competing for focus. In any case, not the stuff on the net is all composed by Moose. Continue to look through the locales until you find not many which are useful. Get your name included in their bulletin records and read up the books they prescribe you to. There is no limit to the degree such data can take care of you. So look into the net and further develop your arrangement today!

CHAPTER 3

LIFTING WEIGHTS: CLOTHES

The vast majority of us will generally be undecided about the sort of garments we will be wearing during our lifting weights practice system. While the puritans in the field underline that the actual system is huge and not the clothing in which it is polished, most others have come to feel in an unexpected way. All types of activities cause a ton of sweat. While practicing for working out we work with a ton of loads, which makes our body sweat bountifully. To guarantee that the tacky dampness doesn't come in that frame of mind while working out, we should wear garments that can undoubtedly retain this abundance of dampness and keep us dry consistently.

Given its simple engrossing powers cotton is the best texture for a wide range of activity wear. It doesn't make any difference what sort of garments you are at last wearing be it a T-shirt or a tank-top or indeed, even a downy shirt, for however long it's cotton you realize you are on safe grounds. Match up these with exercise jeans and you are good to go for your activity program. Jocks, of the two genders, appear to be especially halfway towards tank tops.

Active apparel makers have asserted it to be the most sweltering selling clothing thing among weight lifters. Tank tops arrive in different varieties, and are for the most part modest and in this way a decent purchase. It helps obviously that tank tops permit a nearby perspective on the competitors' siphoned-up muscles permitting them to get a decent look of the sort of headway they are making. Lifting weights has a ton to do with feeling, individuals who exercise don't simply need a fit body they likewise need a lovely body. A tank top permits them to display this hot body. In some cases that there isn't anything more rousing than having the option to see your level-up body in the mirror before you. A tank top makes such a view effectively conceivable.

Regardless of all in addition to focus, there are a couple of weaknesses of wearing a tank top. First off tenacious tank tops will generally keep your body wet and consequently pass up the entire reason for cotton wear. Sticky garments can be a significant issue while working out, subsequently, an especially close tank top ought to be given a miss for a somewhat free one. Besides, various female muscle heads are worried about how much skin a tank top generally will in general show. Wear a tank provided that you are agreeable to it, you would rather not be worried about the thing you are showing when you are focusing on your activity. Then again, ensure you are not wearing something superfluously uncovering, the exercise center is not a wet shirt challenge and a lot of skin can demonstrate diverting for the others practicing around you.

Match your tanks with a decent set of loose track pants; these are open and consequently very agreeable. Most competitors today are inclined toward a casual fit as opposed to the tight spandex fit that had been well known among past weight lifters. There is a scope of such loose exercise center jeans accessible in the market today, they come in different alluring tones and are normally very reasonable.

CHAPTER 4

WEIGHT TRAINING: UNDERSTANDING ANATOMY

To be a specialist weight lifter you should try to comprehend your body's life structures. To construct your muscles satisfactorily you should know precisely where every one of them is found and the way that they may be grown effectively. This could sound simple in any case, it is not a stroll in the park, particularly due to the frequently unpronounceable names of the muscles.

To realize your muscles intently thusly find a mirror and attempt and find each of the muscles on your body all alone. We should start with the neck. In your neck region, there are two essential muscles you can focus on during your lifting weights schedule. These are the upper trapezius and the levator scapulae. The first is the muscle that runs down from your scruff to your shoulder. The last option runs lined up with the underlying cervical vertebrae in your neck.

The trapezius affectionately called the snare muscles move down the scruff of your neck and around the midriff on the two sides of the spine. On your shoulders you will track down the deltoid muscles, likewise called the delts. On the forward portion of the shoulder is the front delt, as an afterthought is the center delt and on the back is the back delt. Simply under the front delt, you will find the rotator sleeve muscles running straight out from the armpit region.

On the chest are your pectorals or pecs. On your arms, you will track down 2 distinct kinds of muscles, the bicep, and the rear arm muscle. The rear arm muscles run down the side piece of your arm from the shoulder till the elbow while the biceps run along within part. The two muscles are very unmistakable on the lower arms. Your muscular strength or abs are found right on your stomach region.

On your legs, you will find the quadriceps muscles or the quads quickly toward the front. The rest of the leg muscles are situated on the back, on your calves for example the lower part of your legs. One more muscle, called the hamstring is situated on your upper leg. However other significant gatherings of muscles remember the glutes for your bum and the lats situated on the upper piece of your back. On your lower back, you will likewise find the lower trap muscles. Very much like a stone worker should know both the material he/she is dealing with as well as the strokes he/she will create on it you, as a weight lifter should likewise know your body (or your material) furthermore, your activity system (or your strokes) unpredictably. Information in regards to both of these fundamental variables is essential for all muscle heads. Except if you know your muscles like the rear of your hand you can not connect with them and foster them satisfactorily.

Consequently, start your lifting weights system with cognizant work to distinguish each of the significant muscles on your body. Focus on each or a gathering of them at a given time. Sort out how you need to shape your body as far as the muscles you want to as needs be practice and approach your exercise.

SORTS OF EXERCISES

You may not know about a portion of the wording utilized in weight training. Along the equivalent line, you ought to understand what certain activities are and how to perform them securely. There are all kinds of activities you can perform - so many, as a matter of fact, space keeps us from posting every one of them. In any case, learning the nuts and bolts can be extraordinary assistance.

Hand weight Bench Press

Sit on the edge of a level seat with the free weights laying kneeling down. In one smooth movement, roll onto your back and bring the free weights up to a position somewhat outside or more your shoulders. Your palms ought to confront advances.

Twist your elbows at a ninety-degree point with your upper arms lined up with the ground. Press the loads up over your chest in a three-sided movement until they meet over the middle line of your body. As you lift, focus on monitoring the loads adjusted. Follow a similar way descending.

Standing Military Press

For this activity, you will utilize a hand weight. Stand with your legs about shoulder width separated and lift the free weight to your chest. Lock your legs and hips and keep your elbows somewhat under the bar. Press the bar to a manageable distance over your head. Bring down the ringer to your upper chest or your jaw contingent upon which is more agreeable for you. This exercise can likewise be performed with hand weights or situated on a weight seat.

Lying Tricep Push

Sit on a level seat holding a twist bar with an overhand grasp. Lie back with the goal that the highest point of your head is even with the finish of the weight seat. As you are lying back, expand your arms over your head with the goal that the bar is straight over your eyes. Keep your elbows tight and your upper arms fixed all through the activity.

The greatest key to this exercise is keeping your upper arms in a decent position. Gradually lower the bar until it nearly contacts your brow. Press the bar back up in a sluggish, clearing circular segment-like movement. Toward the completion, lock your elbows totally.

Side Lateral Dumbbell Raise

Stand upstanding with your feet shoulder width separated and your arms next to you. Hold a free weight in each hand with your palms moved in the direction of your body. Keep your arms straight and lift the loads out and up to the sides until they are marginally higher than shoulder level. Then, at that point, gradually lower them back down to your side once more.

Keep your palms rotated toward the ground as you lift the free weights so your shoulders as opposed to your biceps accomplish the work. Ensure you are lifting the hand weights up as opposed to swinging them up. Try not to incline forward while doing this either or you risk injury to your back.

CHAPTER 5

TEST MEAL PLANS

Picking the correct method for eating to fabricate muscle can be a little overpowering. However, when you start eating the manner in which you really want to, it will turn out to be natural to you. Following is a rundown of good food sources for you to eat in every one of the classes you want to focus on:

Proteins:

White meat chicken or turkey

Canned fish

Canned salmon

New Fish

Shellfish

Eggs

Tofu

Soy

Red meat like steak or dish

Complex Carbohydrates:

Oats

Potatoes

Sweet potatoes, Sweet potatoes, Acorn squash

Rice

Vegetables

Corn

Vegetables:

All water-based types.

Lettuce, Cabbage, Spinach

Asparagus

Bok Choy, Leeks

Tomatoes

Celery

Onions

Green Beans

Broccoli, Cauliflower, Radish

Zucchini Squash

Mushrooms

Carrots

Peas

Meal 1:

Vegetable omelet (3 egg whites, 1 entire egg, 1 cup veggies) You can likewise add some chicken or on the other hand, lean meat assuming you need it.

Meal 2:

One cup of yogurt or a protein shake

Meal 3:

6 oz Chicken

A little crude vegetable plate of mixed greens

1 bagel

Meal 4:

1 piece natural product

3-4 oz Chicken

Meal 5:

6 oz fish

1 - Cup barbecued veggies

1 - Cup earthy-colored rice

CHAPTER 6

GOOD NIGHT (GETTING ENOUGH REST)

Rest is one of the most disregarded pieces of an activity routine, however, actually, it is a very significant guideline. Rest is one of the most important devices for development that you can have in your weight training armory. Muscle transformation and development frequently happen around evening time. During the suspended condition of movement you are in, your body is doing the precisely exact thing you have been requesting that it do during your exercises construct muscle.

The absence of rest can intoxicatingly affect your body. As indicated by the Journal of Applied In Sports Science, being conscious for 24 hours has a similar actual impact as a blood liquor content of 0.096, which is over the legitimate driving breaking point in many states. Resolving in this state has its conspicuous drawback. First off, your absence of solid coordination places you at a lot higher gamble for injury. Similarly, as you'd never go to the rec center in the wake of drinking a couple of brews at your nearby bar, you ought to never work out after not resting the night prior. You're in an ideal situation holding on until the following day when your body has been given legitimate rest.

Weight training For Ladies

Numerous ladies are worried about how their bodies look. Abstaining from excessive food intake and weight fixation are very genuine pieces of life for some ladies. Working out and ladies truly fit together well when you consider it. Zeroing in on solid weight gain and muscle wellness makes a lady look and feel quite a bit improved.

Working out is much more than consuming fewer calories and lifting loads. A significant part of the guidance surrendered past parts can apply to all kinds of people. Be that as it may, ladies truly do have to change a couple of things with regards to an exercise plan that will work. A few ladies have never considered working out as a game since they are anxious about the possibility that they will get huge, cumbersome, and become manly looking. Nothing could be further from reality. A trim, strong body on a lady is incredibly provocative and exceptionally sound.

Ladies can't normally create how much testosterone men do, so it is unthinkable for ladies to expand their muscle size in the same ways that men do by simply getting weight or then again two. Without counterfeit substances, ladies will not have the option to get similar mass as men do. Nonetheless, a significant number of the very exercise counsel that we provide for men apply to ladies too: eat 5- 6 little feasts each day, drink a lot of water and get loads of rest. The exercises are equivalent to well albeit a few ladies might need to restrict their reps at first until their solidarity is developed.

Numerous ladies battle with the overabundance of fat and fat muscle tone on their thighs and in their bottom. Since ladies are normally curvier than men, working these regions makes for an extremely complimenting figure.

CHAPTER 7

YOUR RESOURCES FOR BODY BUILDING

In this, the best data age ever, there are many, many spots you can go to for replies to practically any inquiry you have for lifting weights. Search out this data, what's more, advance however much you can. This will make you a superior weight lifter and a more secure one at that! Regardless, you want to buy into two or three lifting weights magazines. The absolute most well, known include:

Flex

This magazine is viewed as the "book of scriptures" of no-nonsense lifting weights. They do interviews with specialists in the field and deal up some astonishing guidance for both the accomplished as well as beginner weight lifter. Find them online at www.flexonline.com or buy into the paper release for just $29.97 per year for 12 issues.

Nothing can truly contrast with individual exhortation and direction. There are numerous rec centers and wellness clubs that have neighborhood associations committed to lifting weights where you can get tips and train with other people who share your enthusiasm. Make an inquiry or two when you are in the exercise center or organization with others in group environments.

The Internet is one more priceless asset for working out data. In exploring this book, this writer relied upon a few of these sites for data. The following are a couple of you ought to truly look at:

www.bodybuilder.com

This site isn't anything not exactly astonishing. You will find more data than you could have ever expected on this site remembering tips for sustenance, test exercise plans, and ways of planning yourself for rivalry.

CHAPTER 8

HELP YOUR METABOLISM NATURALLY

At the point when we are youthful, our digestion is normally high, yet as we age that simply isn't the case. Do you recall the days when you could eat anything that you needed whenever and never appear to acquire a pound? Those days were a perfect, and distant memory. Anyway, there is trust. Of course, we live in an age when we as a whole need to find a speedy path of least resistance to everything. We need to find an enchanted pill that will change our lives, and the truth of the matter is that there are a large number of them that case to do precisely that.

These pills can be exceptionally hazardous and, surprisingly, dangerous on the off chance that they are not utilized as expected. The upside news is that you don't for even a moment need them. There are numerous arrangements that you can without much of a stretch use to help your digestion in a regular way that won't truly hurt more than great..Everything thing that you can manage is to work out consistently and eat a fair eating routine as coordinated by the food guide pyramid.

Regardless of whether you have an ailment that expects you to have a unique eating routine, you can in any case help your digestion. Part of having decent digestion is having great actual well-being and the other part is having great psychological wellness. Individual wellness is vital in keeping high digestion. This doesn't imply that you must be thin it simply implies that you must be fit. Drinking specific teas like green teas can likewise assist you with detoxifying your body which will likewise help your digestion. Green tea has become exceptionally well known in a couple of years as a method of doing this.

Likewise, it is fundamental that I notice that a protein-enhanced diet will assist you with building up your body's regular bulk too. Adding specific nutrient enhancements can likewise help.you to support your digestion. Nutrients like **vitamin E, D, C, and B** will be perfect for supporting your digestion. If you could do without taking them in pill structure you can track down these nutrients in many foods grown from the ground that are in their most regular state or steamed.

Green vegetables are extraordinary wellsprings of normal nutrients and minerals that your body needs to remain fit and solid. Assuming that you are counting calories you ought to ensure that you are eating adjusted feasts. Getting solid and supporting your digestion ought to remain closely connected. If not, you will just prevail about harming yourself.

The South Beach Diet And Metabolism

The South Beach Diet guarantees that a logically demonstrated program makes certain to help you accomplish your objectives and goals for getting in shape securely. This diet will assist you with getting in shape quickly and further develop your heart well-being simultaneously. By and large, most people lose between 8 and 13 pounds in the initial fourteen days when they start the south oceanside eating routine arrangement.

The South Beach Diet is not the same as the Atkins Diet since it is neither low- carb nor low-fat. All things being equal, the eating routine trains you to depend on the right carbs and the right fats. This process is simplified by utilizing a three-stage process that starts with banishing your desires, and closes with introducing an eating routine arrangement that is intended to keep going forever. The genuine worth in the South Beach Diet is the sound nourishing guidance that you will get. This diet holds the main piece of Atkins' routine, eating meat while forgetting the theory that you can eat low-carb food sources. All things considered, you are urged to eat a well-adjusted diet until the end of your life. This sounds simple, right?

The eating routine of the South Beach plan ought to be made out of a lot of natural products, vegetables and entire grains, nuts, and sound oils. Innumerable individuals from around the country keep on going on and on over about the weight reduction achievement that they have encountered in light of this eating routine. This program is not difficult to learn and incorporate and is becoming one of the most famous types of consuming fewer calories around in light of the achievement rate and dietary opportunities included.

Famous people love the South Beach diet plan and depend on it. That is where a large part of the mayhem came from, yet it doesn't imply that the eating regimen doesn't work. The typical individual views that as this diet as one of the less expensive and simpler ones to keep up with since it requires adjusted eating propensities rather than hardship. Maybe that is the reason so many stays on this diet for eternity.

The South Beach diet offers a lot of assortment to what you can eat and makes it so you can partake in your feasts without feeling hungry. This diet is not difficult to follow and is exceptionally worth the time put resources into learning it. On the off chance that you make it a drawn-out piece of your workout regime, you will notice that you have more energy and your digestion will get the kick-off that you want.

UTILIZING FOOD TO BOOST YOUR METABOLISM

When a large portion of us ponder our digestion it is generally as far as shedding pounds. Our weight and our digestion are what we use to characterize our bodies nowadays. The main issue with this is that we are likewise liable to fail to remember that eating less junk food implies a shortfall of food, yet all at once the moderate admission of food. It isn't solid nor is it brilliant to take on those craze slims down like the Atkins, South Beach, or Zone eats less which compels you to surrender specific food sources because they just work for the length of the time that you are following that eating routine. If you don't proceed that way the weight that you free is all short-lived.

Food is the way to help your digestion and when it comes in its most normal structures, it can likewise, be your best device in keeping an extraordinary load for your body size and type. At the point when I say normal structures I mean for instance when you eat vegetables and organic products it assists with eating them in the structure that they normally come in. on the off chance that you eat organic products from a can, it is contained in syrup and sugars that won't be great for you so eating them crude is the most ideal decision.

At the point when you are eating vegetables, it is ideal to eat them crude and steamed because it keeps all of the nutrients and minerals in them. You ought to likewise keep away from handled food sources and seared meats. Try not to get me wrong, fats are an important part of sustenance anyway, so soaked fats are not. The right equilibrium of food varieties in a day can give your digestion a lift that pills and prevailing fashions can't.

It is ideal to eat no less than three feasts per day that are offset with every nutrition type as recommended by the food guide pyramid in the middle between snacks too. What individuals can be sure of is that it is ideal that you eat five little dinners daily rather than benefit from your metabolic framework. The more food sources that you consume in a day that are sound the better to help your digestion.

It is generally difficult for a large portion of us to follow the food guide pyramid; nonetheless, it is a yet awesome method for guaranteeing that you capitalize on your endeavors. Diet and exercise consolidated is an awesome method for helping your digestion normally, however, if you can't do both strolling and it is the to eat right method for going. There is no genuine reason not to do both, yet referencing them was essential

CHAPTER 9

THE HARM OF USING DIET PILLS

Diet pills, which are likewise ordinarily called craving suppressants, have been endorsed by specialists since the 1950s. At the point when they were first acquainted with people in general, most diet pills contained amphetamine which is also called speed. This medication is exceptionally habit-forming and specialists immediately understood that craving suppressants that contained it wouldn't end up being the momentous weight reduction arrangement they were looking for.

As time passed by, a few different medications, for example, fenfluramine and dexfenfluramine (which are more normally realized by their particular trademarks Pondimin and Redux) went onto the market..Before long thereafter, specialists began joining a medication called phentermine with fenfluramine to shape the now scandalous fen-phen diet pill. Anybody who has focused over the most recent twenty years will recollect how severely that ended up.

Like any remaining medications, weight reduction drugs should be supported by the Food and Drug Administration (FDA) before specialists can legitimately recommend them to their patients. Also as well as endorsing the medications for human use, the FDA is too liable for continually checking the impacts that such meds have on the well-being of the individuals who take them. As a method for managing the consistent requirement for FDA endorsement and guidelines, the dynamic fixing that is much of the time utilized in many eating regimen pills isn't a medication any longer.

All things being equal, these items commonly comprise normally happening spices and are sold without a solution over the counter. Maybe the most famous natural enhancement utilized in diet pills is ephedra which is additionally found to cause significant medical conditions. Green Tea and caffeine are additionally incredibly well-known added substances to most eating routine pills today. Ideally, we will discover that there is just no safe eating regimen pill available. We should all adhere to eating fewer carbs and practice keeping a great weight.

Consuming fewer calories To Boost Your Metabolism

Any individual who is endeavoring to get thinner is constantly told to think about investigating all of the accessible weight reduction diet plans before choosing one. Weight reduction diet hypotheses are found basically wherever you look. The most famous one of the pack seems, by all accounts, to be the high protein and low sugar plan that most dietary specialists use themselves and prescribe to their patients. We as a whole know that the way to shedding pounds lies in your digestion.

The huge accentuation that essentially every reasonable weight diminishing eating routine arrangement ought to be solid weight reduction, not quick weight reduction because a considerable lot of the 'quick' diet plans are undependable or solid. Because of this, the best kind of weight reduction is a calorie-diminished variant of a solid adjusted diet. This diet ought to envelop food varieties from all the different nutrition classes that are illustrated in any food pyramid just to a great extent.

Many specialists and doctors who examine weight reduction are currently beginning to zero in on how low-carb food sources can help individuals attempting to shed pounds. The low starch food sources that are as of now accessible are not normal for all solid bites that have preceded them. They are delicious, and in light of their notoriety, they are modest and can have a prompt effect on how you look and feel.

We as a whole need to get in shape quickly, ideally by eating our ordinary most loved food varieties. Sadly, fruitful weight reduction implies that you need to focus on a sluggish yet consistent weight reduction process. Furthermore, a difference in dietary patterns. The sooner you concentrate on which weight reduction diet plans will work for you, the sooner you and every one of your companions will see the better than ever you. With regards to time to pick the right weight-reduction plan that depends on the food, it is ideal to pick the eating routine arrangement that best relates to the kinds of food sources that you currently prefer to eat since this sort of diet plan will be the least demanding to adhere to. Other than that, they all have their upsides and negatives.

Utilizing Low Carb Diets To Boost Your Metabolism

The low-carb diet frenzy that is continuing right currently is an industry that is picking up speed and request consistently and is making it clear that things are not pulling back. This is an astounding achievement for Dr. Atkins, whose book was quickly named possibly risky at the point when it originally hit the racks a long time back and again after he kicked the bucket.

Presently, every person who views himself as overweight, and some others are raising a ruckus around town searching for whatever might be most ideal high protein and low eating routine food varieties that they can find. The effect of low-carb diets can be felt in about each industry.
A large number of examples of overcoming adversity have individuals going to the rec center at a record rate. They realize that the Atkins and the South Beach Diet will assist them with getting thinner, however, they need to keep that load off as far as might be feasible thus they consequently start to get more dynamic as well.

The central parts in the basic food item industry are currently making significantly more space on their racks to oblige the low-carb food sources. Last, but not least, the low-carb food producers kept on flourishing as their business keep on improving at record levels. The low carb slims down are in any event, beginning to meaningfully affect the menus at drive-through joints. The wraps are entirely great.

Regardless of where you look, low-carb food varieties are ready to move at sensible costs. There could be no more straightforward method for losing those undesirable pounds and keeping them off. Low carb abstains from food are setting down deep roots. It depends on you whether you ought to attempt the low-carb diet, yet assuming that you do, it has never been more straightforward than it is presently. You realize that an eating regimen plan is popular if spots like Subway and McDonald's are beginning to oblige it. Since they drove the way, most other chain cafés are presently doing it also. A portion of the cafés that deal low carb feasts include Applebee's, Arby's, Wendy's, Chi's, and Boston Market Slimming down with low carb admission will assist with helping your digestion however provided that you stay with it as an extremely durable way of life change. What's more, that is its reality. It is more secure that if you decide on this technique you attempt to try not to take any eating routine pills with it. All diets fill their need, yet all the same, the low-carb diet has been known to hurt specific individuals, so make certain to counsel your specialist before focusing on any of them.

CHAPTER 10

LIFTING WEIGHTS SUPPLEMENT REVIEW: EAT RIGHT TO FEEL TIGHT

Lifting weights is a game that requires something beyond the soul to fabricate your body. The utilization of enhancements will assist you with getting another shape altogether. There are heaps of enhancements that you can decide to construct your body. The enhancements can be utilized according to the thoughts that you need to assemble your body. It is the decision of the right enhancement that will have the effect. The most fitting one will help your exercise.

Here is a survey about the lawful and well-known supplements that are utilized to construct the body.

Creatine

Creatine is utilized in numerous areas in lifting weights. This is the enhancement used to add on the bulk and assist the jocks with acquiring strength. Creatine is likewise used to kill the weakness in the jocks after their weighty exercises. It improves the body's digestion and processes food in a superior way and decreases the cholesterol in the framework.

Nitric Oxide

Nitric oxide is utilized to upgrade the exhibition of the muscle-building specialists in our body. It likewise assists you with expanding the weight you lift, and it supports the result, aside from these, it enlivens the course of muscle constriction. Furthermore, it is accepted that nitric oxide improves endurance and sexual sentiments.

Proteins

Protein is given an essential spot in any jock's eating routine. This goes about as the structure block in muscle-building supplements and it assists work with massing in every conceivable manner. This is an amino corrosive which makes a difference in building all around very much conditioned fit muscles. Starches are the best structure to take protein supplements. Whey Protein is one of the quality protein supplements that anybody manufacturer utilizations to construct his muscles in the manner in he needs.

Glutamine

Glutamine is frequently alluded to as the 'attractive sister' of creatine. Incidentally, glutamine is an amino corrosive created by the body normally. It is to be noticed that the degree of regular glutamine found in our body diminishes because of the weight on the body, including the exercise pressure. The shortfall of glutamine would discolor all the difficult work that you did at the exercise center, as it prompts muscle misfortune.

The wellness magazines regularly practice it to survey every one of the enhancements that are utilized in working out. The surveys generally assist the muscle heads by letting them with picking what they need, in light of the sort of body they need. Simply connect for themselves and tone your muscles up.

CONCLUSION

Weight training turned into a frenzy from 1970, for the most part, because of the film Pumping Iron highlighting, no awards for speculating, Arnold Schwarzenegger. While attempting to lift weights, you must think about your objectives first. Is it to fabricate bulk, to shed pounds, or to tighten up?

The hardware you decide to utilize whether at home or exercise center, relies on these variables. The most fundamental need served by working out, as the name recommends, is to foster muscle mass. For this, you want a couple of free loads which, aside from being the best working out gear, are likewise the most affordable. Add to this the way that they are versatile, arrive in an assortment of plans and you know why they sell like hot cakes. Free loads are the most valuable wellness gear as they can be adjusted to your exercise by expanding the load as you get used to your ongoing system.

Lifting weights is likewise a game now and for those keen on preparing for the calling, a legitimate routine in counsel with a subject matter expert and a specialist would be fitting. To the extent that the wellness routine goes, a weight seat with a bunch of free weights from ten to forty pounds is great for building enormous muscles. Simply move gradually up a bit by bit to the heavier loads. For the people who don't need the meaning of the experts, hand weights are the best approach. Simply convenient, one might get a couple of sea-going free weights to rehearse in the pool.

This is particularly for those with back issues and joint pain. Pull-up bars and push-up stands are perfect for conditioning your chest area and arm chiseling, as they take it through the entirety of its speeds. Zero in on regular yet less number of reps for conditioning and serious reps two times or threefold every week assuming that you need mass. Plunge remains then again, give your wrist that additional help and help in fortifying your arms and hands. Whether an expert etc., remember that you want to substitute and enhance your work-out daily practice with satisfactory sustenance and rest.

Weight training is massively burdening, what's more, you want to be careful if you would rather not wind up harming yourself. Although you may need to work out regularly, recall that your body needs to recover between exercises. Contingent on your wellness level, go for the gold five serious exercises each week and step by step increment the power and length of your exercises. At long last, show restraint. Assuming that you have never practiced in your life to date, odds are you will take some time to become acclimated to it. Make an everyday practice, counsel a specialist and a subject matter expert, get legitimate nourishment, and adhere to your routine. Your endeavors will be compensated eventually.

www.ingramcontent.com/pod-product-compliance
Lightning Source LLC
LaVergne TN
LVHW020538160826
845677LV00015B/4129

* 9 7 9 8 8 4 6 2 1 4 2 7 9 *